reflexology

BEGINNERS GUIDE TO ELIMINATE PAIN, LOSE WEIGHT, AND DE-STRESS WITH ANCIENT TECHNIQUES

Disclaimer

The information in this book is not to be used as medical advice and is not meant to treat or diagnose medical problems. The information presented should be used in combination with guidance from your physician.

Disclaimer and Terms of Use: Effort has been made to ensure that the information in this book is accurate and complete, however, the author and the publisher do not warrant the accuracy of the information, text and graphics contained within the book due to the rapidly changing nature of science, research, known and unknown facts and internet. The Author and the publisher do not hold any responsibility for errors, omissions or contrary interpretation of the subject matter herein. This book is presented solely for motivational and informational purposes only.

Introduction

Reflexology is an ancient technique that offers countless benefits to the over-worked and stressed people of the world. The technique is rooted in the simplistic idea of pressure and touch. In our world of separation, it's rare that we ever reach out and touch each other. As a result, we are seeing the dying fruits of our lack of community in our significant influx of sickness, illness, discomfort, and stress.

Foot reflexology brings deep relaxation and therapy to all the organs of your body. Your foot, with all its intricate bones and sensors, becomes a microcosm for the rest of your body. Find a direct link to your head, your neck, your lungs—all the different centers and organs—in order to derive comfort and wellness to these systems. Because of the toxic environment and the preservative-rich diet of our current lifestyles, your body is blocked, imbalanced. Each of your organs is rich with toxins, and these toxins disallow important nutrients to penetrate into your cells to bring you ultimate strength and interior calm.

Reflexology lends complete stress reduction and ultimate relaxation to all parts of your body. It initiates relief to your tense shoulders after long days huddled over a desk, and it regulates your thyroid to yield essential weight loss. Remember that weight loss isn't completely centered on the idea of "calories in, calories out." Instead, you gain weight because of a circulation imbalance, toxic glands, and a de-regulated thyroid. The pounds creep on your belly area because of your increased level of cortisol, the stress "fight-or-flight" hormone. Cortisol also acts as a free radical, killing off cells in the area of your brain called the hippocampus and other cells throughout your body. Your body cannot maximize its potential when you're pulsing with cortisol. Instead, it slowly kills you from the inside.

When you begin reflexology techniques, your body instantly reaps the rewards of enhanced circulation. Better circulation, according to reflexology, yields a better flow of energy. When your body has an ease of energy, your body can boost its metabolism, heal its interior cells, and give you greater amounts of energy. Furthermore, when your body maintains better circulation, your blood can flow more easily to all the cells in your body. Your blood brings necessary oxygen and nutrients to these cells. This prevents cell death and helps your cells to rejuvenate themselves.

Reflexology both cures your interior pains and sends assistance directly to the root of your symptoms. This is different from regular, modern-day medical drugs that work to eliminate your symptoms. These drugs ignore the basic reason for these symptoms, and therefore you cannot find a necessary, ultimate relief for the problem. Your life becomes a series of pills with a lifetime of side effects.

Reflexology techniques look to a basic map of the human body found on the human foot. This book outlines the necessary motions you must utilize to maximize each of the relaxing components of reflexology. Later outlined charts show you where to massage on your foot if you want to send healing powers to your spleen, for example. If you want to relieve yourself of a headache, you'll begin to release the initial tension in the top of your big toe. Each portion of your body is linked to your foot, and you can de-block these portions to bring ultimate relief.

Many people proclaim reflexology as a faux-science. However, recent scientific understanding of reflexology further links your foot with the rest of your body. 19th and 20th century doctors began to utilize the technique to boost health, and current European and Asian doctors administer reflexology techniques alongside modern-day medicine. Reflexology has its place in any person's healthful lifestyle—regardless of your health problems or relative wellness. Everyone needs relief. Everyone needs to be touched. These things are necessary components of a beautiful, healthy life.

Look to reflexology if you are a person with chronic fatigue and never-ending stress. Look to reflexology in order to relieve your interior tension, boost your weight loss goals, and find greater pleasure in the bedroom. Understand how to bring these healthful

components into your daily life and reap the rewards
of the ancient techniques of reflexology.

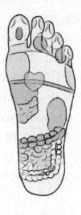

Table of Contents

Introduction 3

Chapter 1: Touch: An Essential Element of Life 9

Chapter 2: Understanding Reflexology 13

Chapter 3: The Ancient Tradition of Reflexology 17

Chapter 4: Myths of Reflexology 21

Chapter 5: Reflexology Charts and Photos 25

Chapter 6: Reflexology Basic Massage Techniques 33

Chapter 7: Reflexology and Stress Relief 49

Chapter 8: Reflexology and Weight Loss 53

Chapter 9: Reflexology and Sexuality 63

Chapter 10: Reflexology and Aromatherapy:
Maximizing Twin Forces 69

Conclusion 75

Chapter 1
Touch: An Essential Element of Life

When was the last time you touched someone? Try to think about it. This morning, you woke up. You rolled away from your partner or spouse onto a cold ground. You jumped into the shower, used a washcloth to cleanse yourself, and leaped into your car to drive to the coffee drive-thru before work. You greeted the person in the drive-thru, and you took the coffee from them without touching them.

You sat at your desk. You had meetings with other professional people, and you reached across the desk in order to shake their hands. There. That's it: your first touch of the day. It is firm, and it is brief. It is meant to be cold and formal, and it brings you no relief from the morning stressors. When you get home from work, do you touch your friends, your roommates, or your family members? Do you hug your spouse? Do you find yourself an island in this world of reluctant touch? Do you find yourself holed up in an age of technology, never seeking the healing abilities of a simple, warm embrace?

Touch is an essential element of your life: one that yields ultimate healing. In our world of spinning machines, humming cell phones, and constant computer screens, our sense of touch has diminished to give way for other, less organic mechanisms for healing. Even doctors utilize machines in order to scan bodies; they no longer look to their hands to aid with their diagnosis.

According to social scientists, if an instructor reaches out to touch a student on the arm, the student is far more likely to exhibit greater participation in class. When athletes reach out to hi-five each other during a game, they formulate a more cohesive team. Why, exactly, does this "touch" resonate with us so much?

Skin is your largest organ and when someone touches that organ, they're contacting pressure receptors called Pacinian corpuscles. This induces pressure stimulation, which sends a direct signal to the brain. This signal targets the vagus nerve, a part of the brain that is connected to different organs in the body, including the heart. When the nerve sends signals to the heart, your blood pressure decreases and your heart slows. When your blood pressure decreases, you are much less likely to feel stress.

When a friendly person touches you, you usually want more. Why is that? Essentially, when you're touched, a region of your brain called the orbital frontal cortex becomes highly activated. This is the same center of your brain that reacts when you eat candy or smell flowers. Your orbital frontal cortex actively "lights up" and rewards you with feelings of joy—the same feelings you feel when you munch on chocolate.

As you begin to learn the benefits of touch and reflexology, try to reach toward your friends and loved ones more often. Experience the sheer joy of a simple hug, and live with the revving orbital frontal cortex, bringing you waves of happiness. The power of touch—even without basic understanding of reflexology—is incredibly clear. Merge yourself with your surrounding world. Reintroduce the power of touch in the midst of thousands of machines and buzzing telephones. Find inner peace.

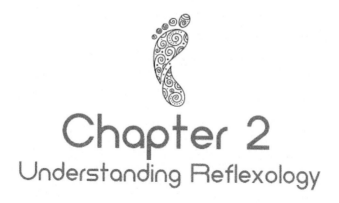

Chapter 2
Understanding Reflexology

Reflexology is an incredible system of massage, of touch, that looks to treat illness and relieve interior bodily tension. It is based on the theory that reflex points on the head, feet, and hands are linked to every element in the body.

Of the head, hand, and foot, the Reflexologist looks to the feet, the mechanisms by which you move from place to place, as the microcosm of the greater human body. This doesn't seem like a far reach. After all: your foot has over 7,000 nerve endings, 107 ligaments, 26 bones, and 19 muscles. Incredible. According to the Reflexologist, the feet represent every organ and every body part. Your two lungs are represented in each foot; your two kidneys are represented on each foot, as well. However, the liver—a singular organ n the body, is represented on the right foot, while the heart is represented on the left foot. In fact, the entire right side of the body is represented in the right foot, while the left side of the body is represented in the left foot. The left foot further presents understanding of the body's past and future.

Whorever an interior organ is represented on the foot, this particular part is called the "uigan roflex." Therefore, where the heart is represented on the left foot, you call this the "heart reflex."

Reflexology introduces a drugless therapy: one that emphasizes the importance of touch in order to provide healing. It looks to alter the body and create a physiological change by improving your body's circulation. Through enhanced circulation, your body reduces its tension and can further create relaxed feelings. Furthermore, this enhanced circulation eliminates your body's waste and restores other bodily functions. Reflexology has been proven to reduce bodily pain and decrease anxiety and depression symptoms. Some proponents believe that reflexology can treat diabetes, cancer, and asthma. It is a completely safe, side effect free treatment that is essential in the betterment of human health.

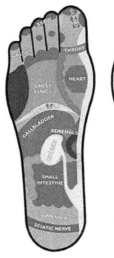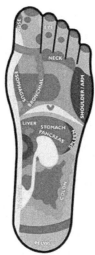

Reflexology Principles

When you begin stimulating the various reflexes on the feet with a massage that emphasizes pressure, the relevant organs in the body become stimulated. When they become stimulated, they begin to heal themselves and unblock themselves. Good blood begins to formulate and bring essential nutrients to these organ cells. Furthermore, the organs begin to detox themselves and excrete poisons that build from poor dietary habits and negative personal thoughts.

This initial body map utilized in reflexology is many centuries old; it stems from a healing circulation that ancient man called our "life force" or our interior "vital energy." According to these ancient techniques, this life force can be supercharged utilizing about eight hundred points in the body. The circulation of

15

energy must flow unimpeded throughout the bodily organs in order to render an intricate balance.

As aforementioned, reflexology works to "unblock" the various organs in the body through pressure in the feet. When one of the organs in your body becomes blocked, the organ actually blocks the flow of energy in your body. It disrupts the circulation and decreases your ability to reach this desired balance. When one organ begins to block energy circulation, the blockage spreads to the surrounding tissues and eventually to the rest of the body. Therefore, if you look to reflexology for immediate direction and balance, you can yield prompt, easy relief from all interior pains. You can create a never-ending balance by targeting the "blocked" organ and disallow this blockage to formulate in the rest of your body.

Reflexology doesn't look to expensive gadgets or never-ending drugs for relief. Furthermore, it's important to understand that reflexologists do not heal people; instead, the body works to repair itself with the relief of organ tension and blockage. Occasionally, the reflexologist can feel the energy move from one part of the body to another. He or she can feel the energy churn from the pressure point on the feet and relocate to the bodily organs. Therefore, the reflexologist and the client can feel the energy flow.

Chapter 3
The Ancient Tradition of Reflexology

Reflexology offers an incredible history that dates back over six thousand years. Foot and hand therapy began in China in approximately 4,000 B.C., and the North American natives were known to practice foot therapy for many centuries to initiate relief.

Ancient Egyptian doctors from four thousand years ago were the first to study the human body on a scientific level. They were able to care for wounds, set bones, and treat a variety of illnesses. Egyptians, some of the first record-keepers, were able to illustrate these dynamic doctor abilities for our later understanding.

A particular pictograph discovered in an Egyptian tomb reveals the third-oldest recording of reflexology. The pictograph is illustrated in the

Saqqara tomb of Ankhmahar. The image of a man working on another man's hand and a different man working on another man's foot reveals the very techniques we practice today. More specifically, the doctors in the pictograph are pressuring the Great toe, known to represent the liver and the spleen, and the thumb, known to represent the lung. Ancient Egyptians respected the body a great deal and seemed to have a higher level of consciousness with regards to it. They wouldn't have popped endless amounts of pills, for example, instead of trying to treat the source of the symptoms.

Present Day Reflexology
Early scientific studies created in the late 19th century paved the way to modern-day reflexology. Sir Henry Head, for example, illustrated the bodily relationship between the skin and the internal organs. Sir Charles Sherrington showed that the nervous system and the body adjust to a particular stimulus when that stimulus is applied to a part of the exterior body. Furthermore, a German doctor named Dr. Alfons Cornellus demonstrated the fact that pressure toward certain bodily spots brings about particular muscle contractions, warmth, alterations in blood pressure, and differences in mental states.

Present-day reflexology finds its basis with two American physicians named Dr. Joe Shelby Riley and Dr. William Fitzgerald. Eunice D. Ingham, of later decades, developed their knowledge in foot reflexology. Ingham has traveled widely in the recent century, yielding her teachings to the world and revealing her method. Recent research validates the true effects of reflexology on many bodily conditions. Chronic conditions, in particular, show dramatic alterations with the utilization of reflexology.

The Chinese government currently accepts reflexology as an undeniable means of curing diseases and preventing illnesses. According to Chinese theory, reflexology studies show that reflexology lends improvement to about ninety-five percent of over eighteen thousand cases. Even Japan and Denmark are hopping on the train, bringing reflexology into employee health programs.

Of course, it's known that stress is growing in our world of constant work and worries. Health problems are linked to these feelings of stress. When the body attempts to function correctly and balance itself in the wake of stress, it falls to illness and damage. With the utilization of reflexology, the body can fall into illness-negating relaxation. The body is able to deal with the various stressors it's up against as the reflexology techniques boost lymphatic drainage and circulation. Reflexology further stimulates the nerve pathways and relaxes the muscles.

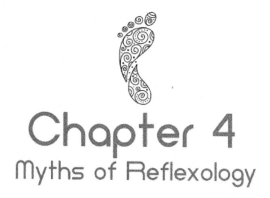

Chapter 4
Myths of Reflexology

Because reflexology isn't rooted in what we think of as "modern" medicine and it doesn't require any synthetic drugs or machines, many people hold myths and suspicions about reflexology. Let's look at the main ones in order to diagnose exactly who should and should not participate in the stunning practice of reflexology.

Myth Number 1: Reflexology is not safe for women who are pregnant.

This is simply not true. If you are frightened of a miscarriage, reflexology can actually help the body to seek necessary balance. Reflexology has never forced the body to imbalance itself and fall into something it doesn't want. Therefore, it has never caused a miscarriage.

Myth Number 2: Reflexology shouldn't be practiced on babies.

Reflexology is actually safe for everyone! Children feel immediate pleasure from pressure on the feet. Reflexologists utilize light pressure for infant feet, and the techniques have been used to relieve illnesses like Colic. Babies enjoy the sensation and are shown to be more relaxed and happy afterwards. If you want to treat your baby without the use of a trained reflexology, try rubbing small areas of the baby's feet with light fingers.

Myth Number 3: People with diabetes should not look to Reflexology.

Again, this is not true. Some people relate reflexology with insulin shock. However, diabetes patients suffer from insulin shock as a result of improper diabetes treatments. This shock is not a result of reflexology. Reflexology should be used to unblock various organs of the body and yield health and nutrients to the cells. It can help with diabetes patients' insulin resistance, as well.

Myth Number 4: Needles are used with reflexology.

This isn't true, either. Needles are used for the ancient technique of acupuncture. Reflexology treatment comes only from the hands of reflexologists.

Myth Number 5: Reflexology is reserved strictly for the feet.

This is not true, either. Reflexology holds benefits when utilized for the face, hands, feet, and ears. Foot reflexology is primarily outlined in this book and is generally the most popular. However, this is because the feet are the most sensitive parts of the body. Usually, hand reflexology is passed down to clients in order to practice their reflexology techniques at home.

Myth Number 6: If you're ticklish, you shouldn't look to reflexology.

This is just silly. When you find yourself relaxing under the touch of the reflexologist, you will fall into the sure and firm touch of the therapy. If you're bracing yourself because you think you're too ticklish, think again!

Myth Number 7: I can't go to the reflexologist after a long day on my feet.

Reflexologists understand how stressful your life is; they can see it on your feet! Therefore, even if you don't have time to "freshen up" your feet before your reflexology appointment, you should not cancel. Your reflexologist will cleanse your feet prior to your treatment using calming essential oils.

Myth Number 8: Reflexology is a sort of myth, a false therapy.

This is not true. Reflexology finds its historical roots in Ancient India, China, and Egypt. Scientists have illustrated its wonderful abilities and the body's incredible energy zone mechanisms for hundreds of years. In 1913, American scientist Dr. William Fitzgerald stated that reflex areas on the hands and the feet were intricately linked to zones in the body. These zones were filled with specific organs. Twenty years later, a physiotherapist named Eunice Ingham built on Fitzgerald's theories and named the mechanisms "Reflexology."

Myth Number 9: Reflexology shouldn't be painful.

Sure. We don't want therapy to be painful. But know that the reflexologist's patients who can handle the pain reap the best interior health rewards from the most painful of techniques. This is because the stronger the technique, the more energy is exerted down the neural pathway of the body to the specific healing organ. Think of it this way: the more energy you put toward something, the greater rewards you reap.

Chapter 5
Reflexology Charts and Photos

Find an extensive list of every organ and every body part represented in your feet. After all, your feet are like a mini model of the human body. As aforementioned, the organs that have a partner or twin are found on both feet; for example, you can find one lung on each foot. For "one-man-show" organs, however, find just one representation on one foot. The liver, for example, is represented on the right foot while the heart is represented in the left foot.

Look to the following charts for a representation of various organs and body parts. Find one of the units of your lungs in the very center of the foot, in approximately the same spot you find it in your own body. See the spleen, where you must massage and exert energy in order to balance your weight loss efforts. Find the heart, where you must exert energy in order to lower your blood pressure. Furthermore, find the shoulders in order to release tension and stress.

Look next to the right foot, in which you find the liver and the gall bladder. See the small intestine toward the inside of the foot, where you must match energy in order to yield nutritive properties to the digestive tract. When you massage the liver and the gall bladder area, you'll secrete the important bile that will break down various fats from recently eaten foods.

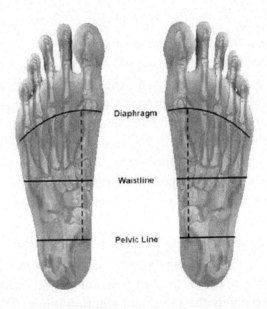

Next, look to the two side-by-side photos of the feet, showing the arms, the lungs, and the breast arena.

Look to the sideways version of the foot for better understanding of the leg, hip, and elbow areas.

Analyze the diaphragm, waistline, and pelvic line segments of the foot. The diaphragm falls about an inch and a half below the line of your toes. The waistline is found right where the first set of toe bones begin, while the pelvic line inserts itself just before the end of the foot, around the heel. Pay attention to these areas because they provide strength to the other vessels of your body.

Foot Reflexology Chart

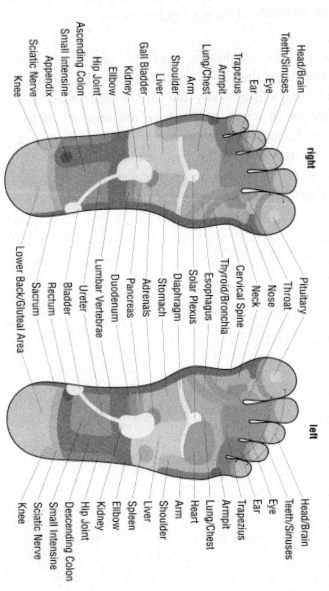

right

- Head/Brain
- Teeth/Sinuses
- Eye
- Ear
- Trapezius
- Armpit
- Lung/Chest
- Shoulder
- Arm
- Kidney
- Liver
- Gall Bladder
- Elbow
- Hip Joint
- Ascending Colon
- Small Intensine
- Appendix
- Sciatic Nerve
- Knee

- Pituitary
- Throat
- Nose
- Neck
- Cervical Spine
- Thyroid/Bronchia
- Esophagus
- Solar Plexus
- Diaphragm
- Stomach
- Adrenals
- Pancreas
- Duodenum
- Lumbar Vertebrae
- Ureter
- Bladder
- Rectum
- Sacrum
- Lower Back/Gluteal Area

left

- Head/Brain
- Teeth/Sinuses
- Eye
- Ear
- Trapezius
- Armpit
- Lung/Chest
- Heart
- Arm
- Shoulder
- Liver
- Spleen
- Elbow
- Kidney
- Hip Joint
- Descending Colon
- Small Intensine
- Sciatic Nerve
- Knee

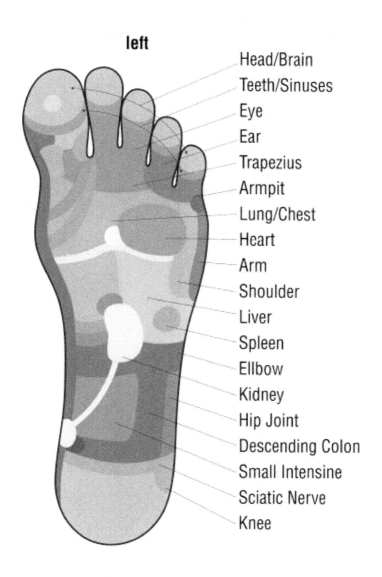

left

Head/Brain
Teeth/Sinuses
Eye
Ear
Trapezius
Armpit
Lung/Chest
Heart
Arm
Shoulder
Liver
Spleen
Ellbow
Kidney
Hip Joint
Descending Colon
Small Intensine
Sciatic Nerve
Knee

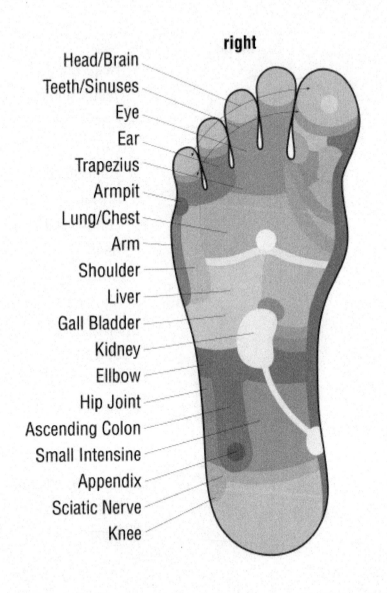

right

Head/Brain
Teeth/Sinuses
Eye
Ear
Trapezius
Armpit
Lung/Chest
Arm
Shoulder
Liver
Gall Bladder
Kidney
Ellbow
Hip Joint
Ascending Colon
Small Intensine
Appendix
Sciatic Nerve
Knee

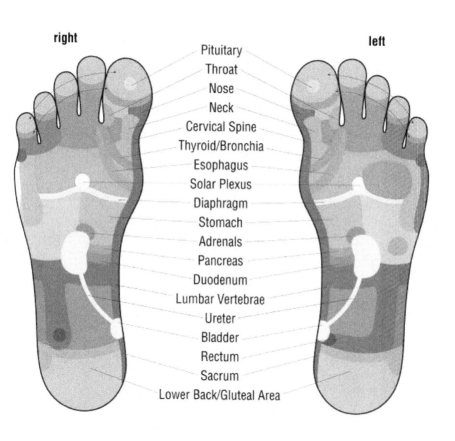

Pituitary
Throat
Nose
Neck
Cervical Spine
Thyroid/Bronchia
Esophagus
Solar Plexus
Diaphragm
Stomach
Adrenals
Pancreas
Duodenum
Lumbar Vertebrae
Ureter
Bladder
Rectum
Sacrum
Lower Back/Gluteal Area

Chapter 6
Reflexology Basic Massage Techniques

Tips and Techniques for At-Home Foot Massage

Foot reflexology is an ancient pressure therapy and therefore involves the application of focused pressure to precise reflex points in the foot. By creating this pressure, the reflexologist can cure and prevent diseases in your body via de-blocking and cleansing your organs. A proper reflexologist can place pressure on various meridians and energy lines on both the side and the sole of the feet in order to discover the cause of your illness. At home, however, you can create some of these initial "wellness" feelings just by doing a foot massage! Read below for better understanding in creating the ultimate foot massage.

Foot Massage Preparation

If you or your partner is giving a foot massage, you must make sure that the foot being massaged is comfortable. Try reclining it on a sofa or a pillow. Utilize some essential oils in these primary moments in order to yield a completely relaxed foot. Allow the foot to be clean and soaked with Epsom salts. Also make sure your feet are completely dry.

INITIAL FOOT MASSAGE TECHNIQUES

1. Stroking

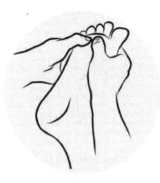

The stroking techniques begin the massage by stimulating foot blood vessels, yielding interior heat. Begin by holding the foot in your hands and massaging the very top surface. Utilize your thumbs and create slow strokes on the top, beginning at the toes and moving the strokes toward the ankles. After your thumbs have reached the ankle, follow this line to retreat back to the toes. You should create a lighter pressure when you're working near the toes because you are dealing with smaller, lighter bones.

2. Ankle Rotation

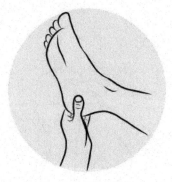

Begin this technique by holding the ankle and moving it side to side in order to loosen the interior joint. Hold onto the heel of the foot with a "cupped" hand, and cling to the ball of the foot with your other hand. Next, rotate the foot first clockwise four times and then counter clockwise four times. When you do this, you will calm the senses.

3. Pivoting

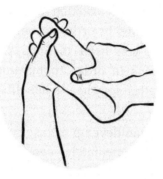

Begin by holding the foot in one hand and utilizing your other hand to gently massage the sole of the foot. Begin the technique in the skin beneath the large toe. Move slowly, using your thumb, to cover the rest of the toes. After you've created the first signs of pressure, roll your thumb back and forth over this skin.

Keep Your Feet Well

Even if you're simply looking to the at-home foot massage techniques in order to enrich your health and happiness, you need to keep your feet well. Follow these tips in order to maximize your foot massage and reflexology health benefits.

1. If and when you develop calluses or corns, do not cut them off. Immediately consult your doctor. Remember that your feet provide a direct pathway to your greater body, and disrupting any element of these pathways could disrupt the entirety of your health.

2. Inspect your feet every day. Watch out for infected toenails, sores, cuts, swelling, and red spots.

3. Always talk to your doctor about your feet if you have diabetes. Diabetic patients have a greater risk of developing foot wound and complications.

4. Always trim your toenails. Cut them straight across and always smooth them with a nail file.

Reflexology Massage Techniques

When you're looking to enhance your interior bodily health, unmask the clog in your body's circulation, and maximize your health, look to the following reflexology techniques. Your reflexology specialist will bring you all the techniques with the proper pressure. However, if you want to practice these techniques at home, you will do no damage. Your body will not correspond with what you tell it via your feet with anything negative.

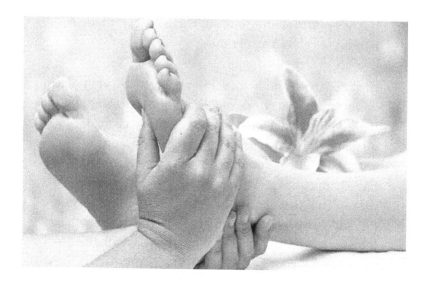

1. Loosen the foot with a Forth and Back Motion

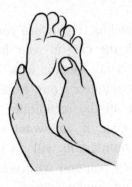

During this mechanism, place both palms of your hands on each side of your foot. Place your fingers on the very top of the foot, and make sure that your hands are relaxed at all times.

Next, push the foot forward slowly with your left hand; at the same time, pull the foot back toward you with your right hand. Invert this mechanism by pushing forward with your right hand and pulling with your left. Maintain a relaxed position with your hands, and repeat this technique approximately six times. You will feel your foot relax beneath your fingers. Next, repeat this process with your other foot. As you enact this technique, you will release tension from your body.

2. The Press and Slide Technique

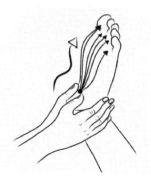

During this technique, you must place both of your thumbs on your heel. Slide the thumbs up from the sole to the very edge of the foot, outwards.

Continue this process all the way up from your sole, toward the middle and then the edge, right before your toes. Always proceed to the edge to bring energy to the outer edges of your foot.

3. Rotate the Toe

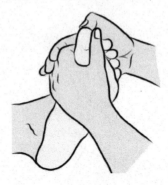

As you rotate the toe, you'll yield a similar feeling of a rotation of the neck. You'll loosen the neck area, and release tension around your skull. This constant nervous tension—a result of your never-ending work schedule, certainly—builds itself in the neck area. Correspondingly, your two largest toes will be very stiff, as well.

Grasp the biggest toe with your thumb and forefinger and twist the toe toward you. Twist it back. Next, create this rotation with the rest of the toes.

4. The Index Finger Technique

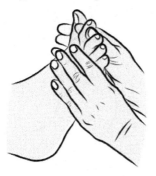

This index finger technique is required when you exhibit energy toward the side and top of the foot. As you make contact with the very edge or the inside of the fingers, always make sure to create a sort of "creep" or slow walk with your fingers.

Keep your pressure completely steady as you "walk" your index finger over a particularly painful reflex in one direction. Work first with your left index finger and second with your right index finger. The joint should only be slightly bent; the inside edge of the finger should bring energy to the appropriate reflex. Make sure not to dig your fingernail into the person receiving the reflexology.

5. The Basic Thumb Technique

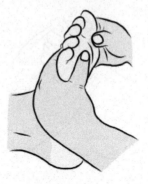

The thumbs are generally utilized to exhibit energy to the soles and occasionally the sides of your feet. Create movement with the first joint of the thumb and creep up on the particular reflex. Do this by bending and then immediately unbending in a sort of creeping "walk." Make sure never to bend your thumb too much so as not to strike the person's feet with your nail.

6. The Hooking Technique

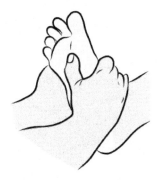

When you "hook," you must support the foot with one hand. This hand is your "holding" hand. The other hand must be placed on the specific reflex area. This is your "working" hand. Hook the thumb of your working hand toward the very outside of the foot.

This allows you to hone in on a very precise, small reflex. You can exhibit energy toward touch-skinned areas of your body, like your heel. When you press your thumb into the particular reflex, you must pull it back almost immediately, like a bee submitting its sting. You must be very precise with this mechanism.

7. Reflex Rotation Technique

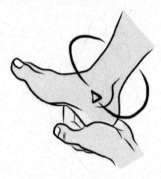

This technique helps you to jostle up and eliminate a particularly painful reflex. You can utilize this technique for the upper abdominal area, illustrated between the Diaphragm Line and the Waist Line. Keep our thumb solid as you come across the particularly tender area and continue to rotate the foot around the "stab" you create with your thumb's pad.

After you continue this rotation for a few minutes, the person will find that the pain has decreased incredibly.

Next, press the "working" hand's thumb into the reflex. Rotate the foot once more with the holding hand: first clockwise and then counter clockwise.

When you create this foot rotation, the nervous system and the blood circulation is enhanced. As your blood circulation is boosted, your nutrient transport from your blood to your organs is elevated. Furthermore, your waste products are skirted away from your body.

Chapter 7
Reflexology and Stress Relief

Causes of Stress

Everyone suffers from feelings of stress. Stress is a necessary element of your physiology. In fact, the human race wouldn't remain alive if it wasn't for stress. Stress produces a hormone called cortisol; this hormone is known as the "fight or flight" hormone. Therefore, when your veins are pulsing with cortisol, you are able to jump higher, run faster, and think quicker. You can pass a big test on a whim, outrun everyone around you in your last leg of a race, and simply live better than you really should be able to—if only for a little while. Your cavemen ancestors were rich with cortisol when predators were chasing them and at least a few of these cavemen ancestors lived to tell the tale.

Your cavemen ancestors, however, always found an easy way to wind down after that first predatory chase. They were able to collect their thoughts around the fire, sleep through the night, and wake up to do it all over again. Stress was not all-consuming like it is now.

Stress Effects

In today's society, stress becomes chronic. When cortisol is in your system for too long, making you stressed throughout every day, your brain begins to fade. Cortisol actually kills some of the brain cells in your hippocampus—or the area of your brain that transfers short-term memories to long-term memories. Because the hippocampus is also the part of the brain that ensures that your brain is creating new brain cells all the time, it's important that you take good care of it. Furthermore, great amounts of continuous cortisol in your system create free radicals in your body that kill cells in all your organs, de-regulate your system, de-balance your circulation, and create poor skin and hair cells. Essentially, stress is the number one cause of inflammation, and inflammation is the number one cause of endless diseases like cancer and diabetes. Furthermore, stress is one of the great causes of our obese society, depositing great amounts of fat in the belly area and increasing waist sizes everywhere.

Stress and the heart—and the risk of heart attack—have an engrained relationship, as well. The more anger, stress, and depression a person experiences, the less that person's heart is able to respond to circulation in an effective manner. The pressure of the consistent emotional highs and lows make the heart stretch too far.

Stress actually depletes your white blood cells and neurotransmitters, as well. This means that stress decreases your ability to maintain health and high immunity. Furthermore, when your neurotransmitters are deregulated, your brain cells have a decreased ability to talk to themselves. When your brain cells cannot communicate, certain things in your body just don't function properly.

Think about the people in your life. Think about which of those people who seem the most stressed, and then think about which of those people get sick the most often. Generally speaking, the people with the greater interior stress reap the greater medical ailments.

Through reflexology, these people can finally seek relief.

Reflexology and Stress Relief

Reflexology brings low-cost relief to the stressed individual. Reflexology treats the body, the spirit, and the mind as a single unit by administering health and energy directly to the cause of the illness and disease. Reflexology actually cancels the effects of stress while bringing balance and relaxation to the body.

When the body is relaxed via the reflexology program, it has a much greater ability to deal with daily living stressors. Reflexology lends a gentle nudge toward greater functionality. It improves the lymphatic drainage and bodily circulation. It further brings muscle relaxation and greater excitement to the neural pathways.

Furthermore, reflexology actually activates various "feel-good" hormones via its stimulation of the lymph circulation. As the circulation is amped, the nerve supply to the cells is increased; this releases toxins from these cells. Furthermore, this allows an increase of endorphins. Endorphins, often thought of in relation to a "runner's high," create an immediate decrease of stressful feelings.

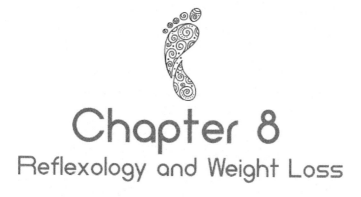

Chapter 8
Reflexology and Weight Loss

Reflexology techniques yield a pleasurable weight loss experience. Specific pressure points on the feet actually trigger interior "weight loss" conducive centers in your body. Look to the following steps to supplement proper dietary restrictions with reflexology. Through reflexology, you can shed the pounds quickly while also fuelling yourself with balance and nutritional health via enhanced circulation.

1. Find your Spleen and Digestive Organ Reflex Points to Decrease Hunger

In order to maximize your weight loss potential, you must find the pressure points on your feet that correspond with your spleen and your other digestive organs. You must massage these weight loss components for about five minutes every single day.

Begin by supporting your left foot with your right hand. Utilize your left thumb in order to massage the "spleen reflex." You can find the spleen reflex on the chart in the oblong area at the very outside edge of your foot. This is between the diaphragm line and the waist line. When you stimulate this area for five minutes every day, you are automatically reducing your hunger.

2. Find the Pancreas and Stomach Reflex Points to Maximize Nutritional Intake

Massage your pancreas and stomach reflex points by holding the left foot with the right hand and exerting effort into the points with your left thumb. When you reach toward the outside limitations of this particular reflex area, it's important that you switch hands and begin to massage the reflex points in the other direction. As you stimulate these points, your body is able to absorb maximum amounts of nutrients from the food you already eat. Therefore, when you eat less food, you'll retrieve the most nutrition from the food you do eat.

3. Find the Gall Bladder Reflex Points to Maximize Weight Loss

Rub at the gall bladder reflex point in order to maximize your weight loss. Your gall bladder stores something called bile. Bile is the digestive juice that your liver creates. This bile emulsifies the fats in your food, and this process increases your ability to lose weight.

4. Boost your Endocrine Glands and Balance Hormones

Look for your endocrine glands in order to create a balanced hormone environment and therefore induce a regulated appetite. Your endocrine glands induce feelings of stress, or the fight-or-flight hormones. Therefore, when you apply pressure to these thyroid reflex points at the very base of your largest toe, you can regulate these hormones. You can further regulate the pituitary gland, which is in the very center of the beginning of the crease in your big toe. Look to the area between your diaphragm line and your waistline in order to pay attention to the adrenals. Massaging all of these areas helps balance your emotions and release stress. When you aren't fuelled with stress, you can pay a lot more attention to your diet. You don't, for example, have to stress and eat an entire box of chocolate. We've all been there.

5. Find your Relaxation Response and Sleep Well

Find the diaphragm line, which is at the external edge of your left foot. Nestle your right thumb across this line. As you do this, bring your toes back away from you and toward you, across your other thumb. When you bend your toes over, bring your right thumb alongside the appropriate diaphragm line. Massage well. This will allow you to avoid insomnia and get a good night's rest; this is essential to allow your body to release the stored fats.

Hand Reflexology for Dieters On-the-Go

The majority of this book centers on the benefits of foot reflexology. However, if you find yourself in the midst of a stressful, packed week, you can look to the benefits of hand reflexology for weight loss and balance.

1. Begin by Finding the Organ and Gland Reflex Points in Your Hand

Find the same pressure points in your hand that you utilize in your feet. Therefore, work with your spleen reflex point, just beneath the little finger on your left hand, your digestive organ reflex point, below the breast and lung center on each of your hands, the gall bladder reflex point, or the pad beneath your smallest finger on your fight hand, and the important endocrine glands, found in the middle of each of your thumbs. Work these centers with your other hands, working up and down and outward for the reflex point.

2. Next, Apply this Pressure Quite Firmly, but Not Painfully

When you find the points you want to press, press them in a deep way. Do not press so deeply that your hand feels pain. However, it's important to exert more pressure on your hands than you do your feet.

3. Play the "Creep" As You Massage

As you press your fingers into your pressure points, creep forward small pieces at a time. Remember to maintain pressure at all times. Remember that your hand pressure points are much smaller and more particular than your feet's pressure points. Therefore, you must work more slowly.

Weight Loss Reflexology Tips

When you're utilizing reflexology to lose weight, you mustn't totally replace your other weight loss exercises and dietary concerns. Instead, reflexology should complement your other work.

Furthermore, you should always get about seven hours of sleep every single night in order to lose weight.

If you want different reflexology tips, look to an ear chart in order to emphasize your ear reflexology experience. Simply find the specific points in the ear that are connected to the spleen, the endocrine system, the gall bladder, etc.

Hand Reflexology Chart

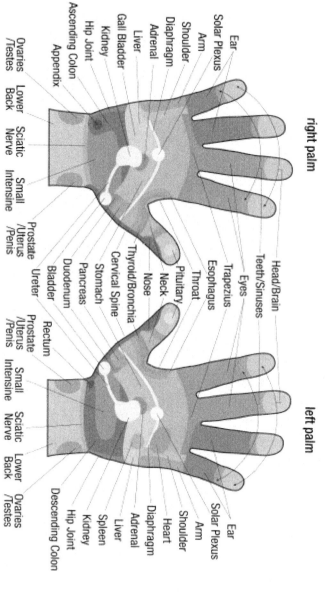

right palm

left palm

Ear
Solar Plexus
Arm
Shoulder
Diaphragm
Adrenal
Liver
Gall Bladder
Kidney
Hip Joint
Ascending Colon
Appendix

Ovaries/Testes
Lower Back
Sciatic Nerve
Small Intensine

Head/Brain
Teeth/Sinuses
Eyes
Trapezius
Esophagus
Throat
Pituitary
Neck
Nose
Thyroid/Bronchia
Cervical Spine
Stomach
Pancreas
Duodenum
Bladder
Ureter
Prostate/Uterus/Penis
Rectum

Prostate/Uterus/Penis
Small Intensine
Sciatic Nerve
Lower Back
Ovaries/Testes

Ear
Solar Plexus
Arm
Shoulder
Heart
Diaphragm
Adrenal
Liver
Spleen
Kidney
Hip Joint
Descending Colon

59

left palm

Ear
Solar Plexus
Arm
Shoulder
Heart
Diaphragm
Adrenal
Liver
Spleen
Kidney
Hip Joint
Descending Colon

Rectum
Prostate
/Uterus
/Penis
Small
Intensine
Sciatic
Nerve
Lower
Back
Ovaries
/Testes

right palm

Ear
Solar Plexus
Arm
Shoulder
Diaphragm
Adrenal
Liver
Gall Bladder
Kidney
Hip Joint
Ascending Colon
Appendix

Ovaries /Testes
Lower Back
Sciatic Nerve
Small Intensine
Prostate /Uterus /Penis

right palm   left palm

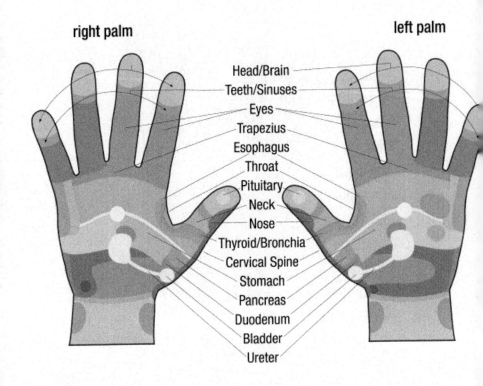

Head/Brain
Teeth/Sinuses
Eyes
Trapezius
Esophagus
Throat
Pituitary
Neck
Nose
Thyroid/Bronchia
Cervical Spine
Stomach
Pancreas
Duodenum
Bladder
Ureter

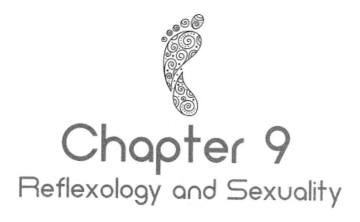

Chapter 9
Reflexology and Sexuality

If you want to rev your sex life, look to the stunning techniques of reflexology. There are several "sex" spots on your feet that stimulate both you and your partner. Reflexology lends awareness of your interior organs, systems, and muscles; it can give you the balance and sex boost your brain and body require.

Find the following areas on your feet in order to maximize your sex life. Alternately, boost your sex life by bringing these reflexology techniques to your partner's feet. Remember that a foot massage pre-intercourse can bring you both together; it can relax you and give you feelings of calm and happiness.

1. Brain

Because you know that the brain influences everything you do in the world—it influences your hormones, your anger, and your happiness—you know you must evoke "sexual feelings" in the brain to maximize your sex life. Find the reflexology foot area on both of your feet. Rub and massage the very fleshy arena of the largest toe. This will immediately enhance your circulation. As your circulation flows, your brain will maintain better communication with your sexual organs. You will have a much easier time of getting "in the mood."

2. Ankles

Look to the very inside and outside of your ankles for nerve-ending heavy spots. These nerve-endings are linked directly to very erogenous zones in your body. Find your reflexology spot to connect to your vagina, penis, prostate, or uterus. Press your thumbs directly in the hollow areas beneath your ankle bones in order to make a connection with these organs. Create small, gentle thumb circles in these hollows to unleash your passion.

On the outside of your feet, in the hollows beneath the anklebones, unleash the reflex connections to the testicles and the ovaries. Massage in small circles in these areas to strengthen your libido, reduce your

PMS symptoms, and increase your fertility.

3. Breast and Chest

The breasts have a large influx of nerve endings, each with a connection in the feet. When you affect these nerve endings, you automatically stimulate the genital area.

Find the connection to your breasts and chest in the soles of your feet. Find this location in the upper middle arena of the sole. Massage here and rev energy waves to your nipples; allow your genitalia to become excited, as well.

4. Stomach

The stomach is one of the most sensual places to touch a person because of the incredible blood flow that occurs between the pelvis and the belly button. When you focus here via reflexology, you can send an influx of sexual energy to your partner.

Find this stomach connection at the soles of your feet, along the interior edge of your central part of the foot. When you massage here with a light thumb, you can relax the stomach, boost circulation, and arouse yourself or your partner sexually.

5. The Back

Think about the shivers you get down your back when you feel amorous toward someone. You feel this because your back is rich with countless nerve endings. When you touch the nerve endings via your reflexology techniques, you can loosen the spine to boost circulation and bring even more of these sexual feelings. Find the link on the soles of your feet, at the interior edge all the way from your heel to your toe. When you pay extra attention to the area from the central part of the edge of your foot all the way to the heel, you can prevent backaches and fuel your chakra sexual energy.

6. Ears

Your ears are pulsing with as much energy as your feet and hands. When you rub your ears or your partner's ears, you can awaken something deep inside. Furthermore, you can lend attention to your ears via a connection in your feet. Find the "ear" on the sole of both of your feet. Press your thumb into the base of the fifth and fourth toes, right on the sole. Open up your ears and begin to communicate and listen to your partner on a different level.

7. Eyes

The eyelids are some of the most sensitive material on your body. If you press on the soles of both of your feet, in the precise area between your middle and second toes, you can improve your eyesight and fuel better understanding between you and your partner. You can see things a bit brighter and heighten your senses.

8. Hips and Legs

These parts of your body, the hips and your legs, are rich with nerve endings that hardly ever see the sun. Find their reflexology counterparts at the exterior edges of both of your feet. Begin the massaging in the middle of the exterior edge. Move slowly toward the heel, formulating tiny circles. When you do this, you can fuel blood to the hips and open up these erogenous arenas.

Clearly, you can influence your sex life via the corresponding locations in the foot. You can fuel your energy—and the energy of your partner—with sensuous massaging and relaxing techniques.

Chapter 10
Reflexology and Aromatherapy: Maximizing Twin Forces

People who practice reflexology state that the marriage of two or more holistic practices and therapies yields a more complete relief from both physical and mental ailments. Most notably, the utilization of aromatherapy to enhance and complement reflexology brings essential healing.

The healing properties of aromatherapy affect the mind and trigger the body's actual healing mechanism. When you inhale essential oils and fragrances, the healing powers enter the bloodstream and activate the olfactory bulb. This yields electrical impulses to the Limbic system, which calms you and alters your emotions.

History of Aromatherapy

The history of aromatherapy dates back several thousand years, much like reflexology. Fossilized pollens found in ancient burial sites show traces of medicinal plants. Ancient man, our ancestors, must have understood which berries, which plant leaves, and which pieces of flowers alleviated pains and aches.

Ancient Egyptians practiced early forms of medicine and much of their work found its roots in plants. They utilized Rosemary and basil, for example, to relieve indigestion and pain.

Furthermore, medieval Europeans utilized plants in pills and potions. They further created nosegays, which were inhaled to fight against pestilence. Lavender, sage, and rosemary, in particular, were used to scent clothing and protect against moths. During plague times, important plants were burned along the streets to disinfect against the plague.

The end of the 19th century brought the aromatherapy discovery by Professor Rene Gattefosse, a chemist of French origin. He discovered that lavender had healing properties when he threw his burned hand into a bowl of lavender oil. After his burn healed incredibly, he began studying the healing properties of other essential oils.

Gattefosse's work was revealed to other French physicians, who utilized essential oils to treat tuberculosis, cancer, and diabetes.

Understanding Aromatherapy

Essential oils are the most powerful, ancient utilizations of therapy in the world. They are extremely concentrated and bring anti-inflammatory and hormone-balancing effects. They help to release pain and muscle tension, and further assist with the overall balance of the body. Aromatherapy produces a better spiritual, physical, and emotional well-being via massaging and inhaling essential oils. These essential oils stem from plants and are chosen because of their specific stimulating, sedative, or refreshing qualities. Aromatherapy does not work to treat the interior body; rather it is meant to treat the mind and bring those feelings of happiness and joy to the rest of the body. As aforementioned, the body is pulsing and stressors that can eventually subside and stop affecting the body.

Rosemary Essential Oil

Rosemary oil lends itself to many Mediterranean dishes and has been utilized for thousands of years for many purposes. Rosemary oil is known to decrease indigestion and relieve stomach cramps. It helps detox the liver and is therefore a wonderful assistant in the art of reflexology, meant to cleanse your interior organs. Rosemary allows your liver to release bile and stimulate blood flow. Through enhanced circulation, the body can create a better balance. Furthermore, rosemary essential oil works as a nerve tonic and is utilized to boost your concentration. It further remedies depression and brain fatigue. It boosts the immune system via the stimulation of antioxidants, and it relieves interior pain.

Basil Essential Oil

Basil essential oils, churned from the seeds and leaves of the basil plant, bring treatment of motion sickness, nausea, diabetes, and constipation. When it's smelled, you feel immediate release of mental fatigue, nervous tension, migraines, and melancholy. You can build your mental clarity and strength. Furthermore, basil essential oils yield essential blood circulation and allow your body to fuel metabolic functions. Through this boost in circulation, your body can balance itself and retain normalcy once more.

Chamomile Essential Oil

Chamomile essential oil comes from a daisy-like plant. It is pulsing with apigenin, which has been shown to fight back against cancer cells in the body. It further boasts alpha-bisabolol, which holds anti-inflammatory and anti-sepctic properties. The chemicals of the essential oil actually bind to GABA receptors; through this binding, you are fueled with feelings of wellness and happiness. When you drink alcohol, chemicals bind with your GABA receptors, as well; therefore, the first feelings you experience when you drink your after-work pint—those feelings of relaxation—are the very ones you experience when you administer yourself with chamomile essential oils.

Jasmine Essential Oil

Jasmine essential oils, coming straight from the jasmine flower, are known to be aphrodisiac in nature; therefore, they decrease your stress levels and put you "in the mood." Sexual activity churns well-being and further brings those essential "touch" benefits noted previously. Furthermore, jasmine is known as an anti-depressant and an anti-septic. The smell releases the hormone serotonin, which elevates your mood and gives you feelings of happiness. Jasmine also lends you undisturbed periods of restful sleep. It reduces your insomnia and allows you to be patient and productive in your waking life.

Combination of Reflexology and Aromatherapy

The combination of reflexology with aromatherapy reveals an extensive, dual therapy program. The aforementioned reflex points are essential neural pathways to bodily organs and blood vessels.

Therefore, the effects of the oils are boosted through this neural pathway in order to vitalize the organs. The reflexology "unblocks" the organs, and the essential oils yield incredible healing properties. This allows the body to find stunning self-healing and natural abilities.

The mind and the body are able to thrive with the marriage of aromatherapy and reflexology. Drop about two drops of the essential oil of your choice on a particular part of your foot in order to achieve unblocking, healing effects in less than two minutes. The essential oils are dropped on this contact point, and their energies are released through electrical impulses. This electrical current runs through the neural pathways in order to unclog the toxic-rich organ in your body.

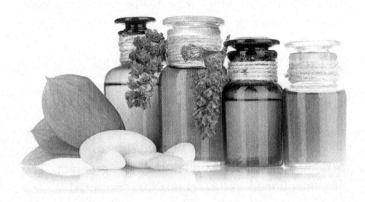

Conclusion

Ancient Egyptian and Chinese reflexology techniques find their necessary utilization in our modern world. As we rush around, stressed and tense, wary of other people's touch, we are killing ourselves. We are reaping the rewards of our materialistic society only to a point, and then we are experiencing un-ending pain. We pop synthetic pills and we find no ultimate relief. Current Chinese and European societies, however, reap the rewards of reflexology alongside modern-day medicines. They understand the benefits of a de-stressed society, and they incorporate the lessons of reflexology.

Look to the necessary benefits of touch in order to enhance your life and find true healing. Learn how to massage the great microcosm of your foot in order to build a connection between your foot, its neural pathways, and its essential life force in your various organs. Create better interior circulation and yield a vibrant energy flow. De-block your organs from the environmental and dietary toxins that they currently contain.

With the refined, ancient reflexology techniques, you can finally relieve yourself of stress. You can create intimate connections with your thyroid in order to build a better, weight-loss-capable metabolism and you can finally shed the pounds you gained from your stressed lifestyle. You can boost your sex life by looking to your sex organs via their representation on your feet and you can administer this relief to your partner, as well. Your life is waiting for you. Relief is waiting for you. Reach out into the world and retrieve the power of touch.

CPSIA information can be obtained
at www.ICGtesting.com
Printed in the USA
LVOW01s1117131215
466478LV00023B/1076/P